TABLE OF CONTENTS

Introduction

If you are wondering about treatment for kidney failure and how kidney transplants work, this concise book is for you. It discusses the following topics:

- Kidney failure
- Treatment for Kidney Failure Options
- What are the basics about hemodialysis
- What are the pros and cons of in-center dialysis and home hemodialysis?
- What questions should I ask about hemodialysis?
- Peritoneal dialysis for kidney failure
- What are the pros and cons of CAPD and automated peritoneal dialysis
- What questions should I ask about peritoneal dialysis?
- Does dialysis cure kidney failure?
- Basics about kidney transplant
- Pros and cons of a kidney transplant
- Questions you should ask about kidney transplant
- Basics about conservative management
- Pros and cons of conservative management
- Can I eat the same foods with any kidney failure treatment?
- How can I decide which treatment is right for me?

- What is the process for getting a kidney transplant?
- Have your kidney transplant
- Who is on my transplant team?
- How will I feel after my transplant?
- How do I know my new kidney is working?

- What are the possible problems after a kidney transplant?
- What are the symptoms of transplant rejection?
- What are the side effects of anti-rejection medicines?
- What should I eat or avoid eating with a kidney transplant?
- And more.

SECTION 1: KIDNEY FAILURE TREATMENT

As your kidney disease gets worse, your health care provider may talk with you about preparing for kidney failure. Talking early with your provider about your treatment options—and making a choice before you need any one of these treatments—helps you take charge of your care. Treatment for kidney failure will help you feel better and live longer.

Understanding the treatment you choose and getting used to the idea that you need this treatment takes time. Each type of treatment for kidney failure has pros and cons. Your choice of treatment will have a big effect on your daily life. By learning about the differences among treatment options, you can choose the one that will be best for you. The more you know about the types of treatment, the better prepared you may be to make a choice.

Learning About Treatment for Kidney Failure

Start learning early about treatment options before you need one. You'll have time to:

- learn about the different treatment options
- talk with other people who are living with dialysis, a transplant, or conservative management
- share your thoughts with your family and loved ones so they can learn about your treatment choices too
- work with your health care team to create a kidney failure treatment plan
- prepare yourself mentally and physically for the changes ahead

Creating a treatment plan and sharing it with your family gives you more control.

Treatment for Kidney Failure Options

You can choose one of three treatment options to filter your blood and take over a small part of the work your damaged kidneys can no longer do. A fourth option offers care without replacing the work of the kidneys. None of these treatments will help your kidneys get better. However, they all can help you feel better.

- Hemodialysis uses a machine to move your blood through a filter outside your body, removing wastes.
- Peritoneal dialysis uses the lining of your belly to filter your blood inside your body, removing wastes.
- Kidney transplant is surgery to place a healthy kidney from a person who has just died, or from a living person, into your body to filter your blood.
- Conservative management treats kidney failure without dialysis or a transplant. You'll work with your health care team to manage symptoms and preserve your kidney function and quality of life as long as possible.

Doing well with kidney failure is a challenge, and it works best if you:

- stick to your treatment schedule.
- review your medicines with your health care provider at every visit. You are the only one who knows how your body is responding to each of your medicines. It's really important that your provider knows which medicines you are taking.
- follow a special eating plan.
- are active most days of the week.

What are the basics about hemodialysis?

Hemodialysis can replace part of your kidney function. In hemodialysis, your blood goes through a filter outside your body and filtered blood is returned to your body. Hemodialysis treatment for kidney failure:

- filters your blood to remove harmful wastes and extra fluid
- helps control blood pressure
- helps balance important minerals, such as potassium, sodium, and calcium in your blood

Hemodialysis isn't a cure for kidney failure, but it can help you feel better and live longer. You will also need to change what you eat, take medicines, and limit the amount of water and other liquids you drink and get from food.

Before you can start hemodialysis, you'll need to have minor surgery to create a vascular access, a place on your body where you insert needles to allow your blood to flow from and return to your body during dialysis.

You can have hemodialysis at a dialysis center or in your home. Hemodialysis is usually done at a dialysis center three times a week, with each session lasting about 4 hours.

Before you can start hemodialysis, you'll need to have minor surgery to create a vascular access, a place on your body where you insert needles to allow your blood to flow from and return to your body during dialysis.

You can have hemodialysis at a dialysis center or in your home. Hemodialysis is usually done at a dialysis center three times a week, with each session lasting about 4 hours.

What are the pros and cons of in-center dialysis and home hemodialysis?

Pros: Dialysis Center

- Dialysis centers are widely available in many parts of the country.
- Trained health care providers are with you at all times and help provide the treatment.

- You can get to know other people with kidney failure who also need hemodialysis.
- You don't have to have a trained partner or keep equipment in your home.

Cons: Dialysis center

- The center arranges treatments, so your schedule is less flexible.
- You must travel to the center for treatment.
- A longer time between treatments means you will have the strictest limits on diet and liquids— because wastes and extra fluid can build up in your body. Having too much fluid in your blood can raise blood pressure and stress your heart. Removing too much fluid too fast during standard hemodialysis also can stress the heart.
- You may have more "ups and downs" in how you feel from day to day because of the longer time between treatments.
- Feeling better after a treatment may take a few hours.

Pros: Home hemodialysis

- You gain a sense of control over your treatments.
(a) You can choose what time to have the treatment; however, you should follow your doctor's orders about how many times a week you need treatment.
(b) You don't have to travel to a dialysis center.
(c) The flexible schedule makes it easier to work outside the home.
(d) You can travel with a hemodialysis machine or arrange for in-center treatment at your destination.

- You'll have fewer "ups and downs" in how you feel from day to day because of more frequent treatments.
- You'll have fewer limits on diet and liquids because the shorter time between sessions prevents waste and extra fluid buildup.
- You can spend more time with loved ones and doing other things because you don't have to go to the dialysis center three times a week.

Cons: Home hemodialysis

- Not all dialysis centers offer home hemodialysis training and support.
- You and a family member or friend will have to set aside several weeks for training.
- Helping with treatments may be stressful for your treatment partner.
- You need space at home to store the hemodialysis machine and supplies.
- You'll need to learn to put dialysis needles into your vascular access.
- Medicare and private insurance companies may limit the number of home hemodialysis treatments they will pay for. Few people can afford the costs for additional treatments.

What questions should I ask about hemodialysis?

You may want to ask your health care provider these questions:

- Is hemodialysis treatment for kidney failure the best treatment choice for me? Why?
- If I'm treated at a dialysis center, can I go to the center of my choice and what should I look for in a dialysis center?
- What does hemodialysis feel like?
- How will hemodialysis affect my [blood pressure, diabetes, other conditions]?
- Is home hemodialysis available in my area? What type of training will I need? Who will train my partner and me?
- Will I be able to keep working? Can I have treatments at night? Will I be able to care for my children?
- How much should I exercise?
- Who do I contact if I have problems?
- Who will be on my health care team? How can the members of my health care team help me?
- Who can I talk with about finances, sex, or family concerns?
- Can I talk with someone who is on dialysis?
- Etc.

Peritoneal Dialysis Treatment for Kidney Failure

Peritoneal dialysis treatment for kidney failure uses the lining of your belly to filter wastes and extra fluid from your body. This lining, called the peritoneum, surrounds your abdominal cavity and replaces part of your kidney function.

You'll need to have minor surgery a few weeks before you start peritoneal dialysis. A doctor will place a soft tube, called a catheter, in your belly. The catheter stays in your belly permanently.

When you start peritoneal dialysis, you'll empty a kind of salty water, called dialysis solution, from a plastic bag through the catheter into your belly. When the bag is empty, you can disconnect your catheter from the bag so you can move around and do your normal activities.

While the dialysis solution is inside your belly, it soaks up wastes and extra fluid from your body. After a few hours, you drain the used dialysis solution through another tube into a drain bag. You can throw away the used dialysis solution, now filled with wastes and extra fluid, in a toilet or tub. Then you start over with a fresh bag of dialysis solution. The process of emptying the used dialysis solution and refilling your belly with fresh solution is called an exchange.

You can choose which type of peritoneal dialysis will best fit your life.

- Continuous ambulatory peritoneal dialysis (CAPD) - An exchange takes about 30 to 40 minutes, and most people need to do four exchanges per day. You sleep with solution in your belly at night.
- Automated peritoneal dialysis, which uses a machine called a cycler to do three to five exchanges per night while you sleep. You may have to do one exchange during the day without the machine.

You may need a combination of CAPD and automated peritoneal dialysis if you weigh more than 175 pounds or if your peritoneum filters wastes slowly. For example, some people use a cycler at night and perform one exchange during the day. Others do four exchanges during the day and use a mini-cycler to perform one or more exchanges during the night. You'll work with your health care team to find the best schedule for you.

What are the pros and cons of CAPD and automated peritoneal dialysis?

With either CAPD or automated peritoneal dialysis, you gain a sense of control over your treatments and don't need the help of a partner. After you're trained, you can do CAPD and automated peritoneal dialysis by yourself. With peritoneal dialysis, you'll have boxes of dialysis solution taking up space in your home.

CAPD pros

- You don't need a machine to do CAPD.
- You can do CAPD at the times you choose, as long as you complete the required number of exchanges each day.
- You can do CAPD in many locations.
- You can travel as long as you bring dialysis supplies with you or have them delivered to where you're going.

CAPD cons

- CAPD can disrupt your daily routine.
- CAPD is a continuous treatment, and you need to do all exchanges 7 days a week.

Automated peritoneal dialysis pros

- You can do exchanges at night while you sleep.
- You may not have to perform exchanges during the day.

- You can travel as long as you bring dialysis supplies with you or have them delivered to where you're going.

Automated peritoneal dialysis cons

- You need a machine. If you travel, you may have to carry your cycler with you.
- Your connection to the cycler limits your movement at night.

What Questions Should I Ask About Peritoneal Dialysis?

You may want to ask your health care provider these questions:

- Is peritoneal dialysis the best treatment choice for me? Why? If yes, which type is best?
- What type of training do I need, and how long will it take?

- What does peritoneal dialysis feel like?
- How will peritoneal dialysis affect my [blood pressure, diabetes, other conditions]?
- Will I be able to keep working?
- Will I be able to care for my children?
- How much should I exercise?
- Where do I store supplies?
- How often do I see my doctor?
- Who will be on my health care team? How can the members of my health care team help me?
- Who do I contact if I have problems?
- Who can I talk with about finances, sex, or family concerns?
- Can I talk with someone who is on peritoneal dialysis?

Does dialysis cure kidney failure?

No. Even when very well done, dialysis only replaces part of your kidney function. Hemodialysis and peritoneal dialysis allow people with kidney failure to feel better and continue doing the things they enjoy, but neither replaces all of the jobs that healthy kidneys do. Over the years, kidney disease can cause other problems, such as heart disease, bone disease, arthritis, nerve damage, infertility, and malnutrition. These problems won't go away with dialysis; however, doctors now have new and better ways to prevent or treat them. You should discuss these problems and their treatments with your doctor.

When do I have to start dialysis?

For most people, the need for dialysis comes on slowly. Symptoms, such as losing your desire to eat and losing muscle, may begin so slowly that you don't notice them. Many people start dialysis when their kidney function (glomerular filtration rate) is between 5 and 10. When kidney function is this low, you may have symptoms from kidney failure and starting dialysis may help relieve them. Starting dialysis treatment for kidney failure can help you regain your appetite and maintain your strength, which is harder to rebuild than it is to retain. Your health care provider can help you decide the best time to begin treatment.

What are the basics about kidney transplant?

Kidney transplant is surgery to place a healthy donor kidney into your body. A working, transplanted kidney does a better job filtering wastes and keeping you healthy than dialysis, but it still isn't a cure.

When you have a transplant, surgeons usually leave your old kidneys in place and connect the donated kidney to an artery and a vein in your groin. The surgeon also transplants the ureter from the donor to let urine flow from your new kidney into your bladder. The transplanted kidney takes over the job of filtering your blood.

Your body normally attacks anything it sees as foreign, so to keep your body from attacking the donor kidney, you will need to take immunosuppressants, also called anti-rejection medicines. Like all strong medicines, anti-rejection medicines have side effects.

A transplant center can place you on the waiting list for a donor kidney if you have permanent kidney damage and your kidney function is 20 or less. While you're waiting for a kidney transplant, you may need to start dialysis.

What are the pros and cons of a kidney transplant?

Together, you and your transplant team should weigh the pros and cons of a kidney transplant.

Pros

- A transplanted kidney works like a healthy kidney.

- If you have a living donor, you can choose the time of your operation.
- You may feel healthier and have a better quality of life.
- You'll have fewer diet restrictions.
- You won't need dialysis.
- People who get a donated kidney have a greater chance of living a longer life than those who stay on dialysis.

Cons

- A kidney transplant requires surgery, which involves   certain risks, such as infection.
- You'll go through extensive medical testing at the transplant clinic.
- You may need to wait years for a donor kidney.
- Your body may reject the donor kidney, so one transplant may not last a lifetime.
- You'll need to take anti-rejection medicines—which may cause other health problems—for as long as the transplanted kidney works.

What questions should I ask about kidney transplant?

You may want to ask your doctor these questions:

- Is transplantation the best treatment choice for me? Why?
- What are my chances of having a successful transplant?
- How do I find out whether a family member or friend can donate?
- What are the risks to a family member or friend who donates?
- If a family member or friend does not donate, who will place me on a waiting list for a kidney?
- How long will I have to wait?
- How will I know if my donor kidney is working?
- How long does a transplanted kidney last?
- What are the side effects of   anti-rejection medicines?

- Who will be on my transplant team? How can the members of my transplant team help me?
- Who can I talk with about finances, sex, or family concerns?
- Can I talk with someone who is living with a kidney transplant?

What are the basics about conservative management?

Conservative management treatment for kidney failure means that your health care team continues your care without dialysis or a kidney transplant. The focus of care is on your quality of life and symptom control. The decision to start dialysis is yours. For most people, dialysis may extend and improve quality of life. For others who have serious conditions in addition to kidney failure, dialysis may seem like a burden that only prolongs suffering.

You have the right to decide how your kidney failure will be treated. You may want to speak with your family, doctor, counselor, or renal social worker, who helps people with kidney disease, to help you make this decision. If you decide not to begin dialysis treatments, you may live for a few weeks or for several months, depending on your health and your remaining kidney function. Many of the complications of kidney failure can be treated with medicines, but only dialysis or transplant can filter wastes from your blood.

As your kidney function declines, you may want to consider adding hospice, or end-of-life, care. You can have hospice care in a facility or at home. The hospice program is designed to meet end-of-life physical and emotional needs. Hospice care focuses on relieving pain and other symptoms.

Whether or not you choose to use hospice, your doctor can give you medicines to make you more comfortable. Your doctor can also give you medicines to treat the problems of kidney failure, such as anemia or weak bones. You may restart dialysis treatment for kidney failure if you change your mind.

What are the pros and cons of conservative management?

The pros and cons of conservative management depend on your current health status. Weigh the pros and cons with the help of your doctor.

What questions should I ask about conservative management?

If you're thinking about conservative management as a treatment for kidney failure, you may want to ask your doctor these questions:

- Is conservative management a treatment option for me to consider?
- Will dialysis improve my quality of life?
- Will dialysis prolong my life?
- Is there any downside to trying dialysis first?
- What should I do to prepare for conservative management?

- Who will continue to provide my care?
- Who will help my family? How long will I live?
- Will I be in pain?
- Can I stay at home?
- Where can I learn more about hospice?
- Who can I talk with about finances, advanced directives, sex, or family concerns?

Can I eat the same foods with any kidney failure treatment?

All of the treatment options for kidney failure require changes and limit what you may eat and drink.

Hemodialysis

Hemodialysis treatment for kidney failure has the most restrictions. You will need to watch how much water and other liquids you get from food and drinks. You will also need to avoid getting too much sodium (a part of salt), potassium, and phosphorus.

You may find it difficult to limit phosphorus because many foods that are high in phosphorus also provide the protein you need. Hemodialysis can remove protein from your body, so you will need to eat foods with high-quality protein such as meat, fish, and eggs. Avoiding foods such as beans, peas, nuts, tea, and colas will help you limit your phosphorus. You may also need to take a pill called a phosphate binder with your meals. Phosphate binders keep phosphorus in your food from entering your bloodstream. Talk with your dialysis center's dietitian to find a hemodialysis meal plan that works for you.

Peritoneal dialysis

Like hemodialysis, peritoneal dialysis treatment for kidney failure requires limits on sodium and phosphorus. You may need to take a phosphate binder. The liquid limitations in peritoneal dialysis may not be as strict as those for hemodialysis. In fact, you may need to drink more water and other liquids if your peritoneal dialysis treatments remove too much fluid from your body. Peritoneal dialysis removes potassium from the body, so you may need to eat potassium-rich foods such as potatoes, tomatoes, oranges, and bananas. However, you'll have to be careful not to eat too much potassium because it can cause an unsteady heartbeat. Peritoneal dialysis removes even more protein than hemodialysis, so eating foods with high-quality protein will be important. You may need to limit calories because your body will absorb sugar from the dialysis solution.

Kidney transplantation

Kidney transplantation has the fewest restrictions on your diet. You will need to limit sodium because it can raise your blood pressure. Medicines that you take after the transplant can cause you to gain weight, so you may need to limit calories.

Conservative management

The diet for conservative management limits protein.

Protein breaks down into waste products the kidneys must remove. Limiting protein may reduce the amount of work the kidneys have to do so they will last longer.

How can I decide which treatment is right for me?

Choosing the treatment for kidney failure that is best for you may be hard. To make it easier:

- start learning about your treatment options early
- think about how each treatment will affect your daily routine and how you feel

Talk with your doctor and with people who are on hemodialysis or peritoneal dialysis, or who've had a transplant, to find out the pros and cons of each treatment. Find out how the treatment changed their lives and the lives of those closest to them. Ask your doctor about the transplant waiting list and about diet changes and medicines you'll need with each treatment.

If you're thinking about conservative management, ask your doctor how you'll feel and how treatment can help keep you comfortable.

Reflect on what's most important to you. If you plan to keep working, think about which treatment can make that easier. If spending time with family and friends means a lot to you, ask which treatment would give you the most free time. Find out which treatment would give you the best chance of feeling good and living longer.

You may wish to speak with your family, friends, health care team, spiritual advisor, or mental health counselor as you decide.

Can I stop or change my treatment once I start?

Yes. You can change your mind. If you don't like your treatment choice, talk with your health care provider about trying something else.

What are some ways to pay for kidney failure treatment?

Medicare, the federal health insurance program, and private health insurance cover most of the cost. Medicare covers kidney failure no matter what your age. If you need more help to pay for treatment, state Medicaid programs provide funds for health care based on financial need. Your social worker can help you find more ways to pay for treatment.

What is an advance directive, and why would I want to prepare one?

You can make your treatment plans and wishes clear to health care providers and family members with an advance directive. During a medical crisis, you might not be able to tell your health care team and loved ones how you want to be treated or cared for. An advance directive is a written legal statement or document with your instructions either to provide or not provide certain treatments, such as dialysis, depending on what else is happening with your health. Advance directives may include:

- a living will
- a durable power of attorney for health care decisions
- a do-not-resuscitate (DNR) order

Living will

A living will is a document that describes the conditions under which you would want to refuse treatment. You may state that you want your health care team to do everything possible to keep you alive, or you may request that they stop treatment, such as dialysis, if you fall into a coma from which you most likely won't wake up. In addition to dialysis, you may choose or refuse the following treatments to keep you alive:

- cardiopulmonary resuscitation (CPR)
- feedings through a tube in your stomach

- use of a machine to help you breathe
- medicines to treat infections surgery
- receiving blood

Refusing to have CPR is the same as a DNR order. If you choose to have a DNR order, your doctor will place the order in your medical chart.

Durable power of attorney for health care decisions

A durable power of attorney for health care decisions, or a health care proxy, is a document that names a person you choose to make health care decisions for you if you cannot make them for yourself. Make sure the person you name understands your values and will follow your instructions.

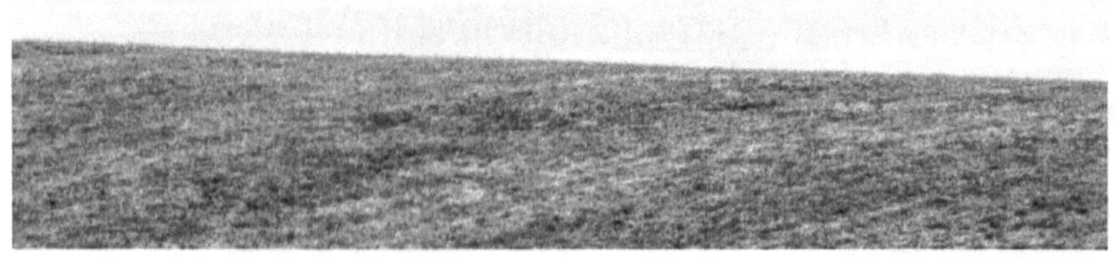

SECTION 2: KIDNEY TRANSPLANTS

KIDNEY TRANSPLANT: HOW IT WORKS

Some people with kidney failure may be able to have a kidney transplant. During transplant surgery, a healthy kidney from a donor is placed into your body. The new, donated kidney does the work that your two kidneys used to do.

The donated kidney can come from someone you don't know who has recently died (deceased donor), or from a living person - a relative, spouse, or friend. Due to the shortage of kidneys, patients on the waiting list for a deceased donor kidney may wait many years.

A kidney transplant is a treatment for kidney failure; it's not a cure. You will need to take medicines every day to make sure your immune system doesn't reject the new kidney. You will also need to see your health care provider regularly.

A working transplanted kidney does a better job of filtering wastes and keeping you healthy than dialysis. However, a kidney transplant isn't for everyone. Your doctor may tell you that you're not healthy enough for transplant surgery.

What is the process for getting a kidney transplant?

If you want a kidney transplant, the process includes these steps:
- Tell your doctor or nurse you want to have a kidney transplant.
- Your doctor will refer you to a transplant center for tests to see if you're healthy enough to receive a transplant. Living donors need to be tested to make sure they're healthy enough to donate a kidney.
- If you don't have a living donor, you'll be placed on a waiting list to receive a kidney. You'll have monthly blood tests while you wait for a kidney.

- You must go to the hospital to have your transplant as soon as you learn a kidney is available. If you have a living donor, you can schedule the transplant in advance.

Talk with your doctor

The first step is to talk with your doctor to find out whether you're a candidate for a transplant. If you're on dialysis, your dialysis team will also be part of the process. If you and your doctor think a kidney transplant is right for you, your doctor will refer you to a transplant center.

Get tested at a transplant center

At the transplant center, you'll meet members of your transplant team. You'll have tests to make sure you're a good candidate for transplant.

Tests will include blood tests and tests to check your heart and other organs—to make sure you're healthy enough for surgery. Some conditions or illnesses could make a transplant less likely to succeed, such as cancer that is not in remission, or current substance abuse.

You'll also have tests to check your mental and emotional health. The transplant team must be sure you're prepared to care for a transplanted kidney. You'll need to be able to understand and follow a schedule for taking the medicines you need after surgery.

In a process called cross-matching, the transplant team tests the donor's blood against your blood to help predict whether your body's immune system will accept or reject the new kidney.

If a family member or friend wants to donate a kidney and is a good match, that person will need a health exam to make sure he or she is healthy enough to be a donor. If you have a living donor, you don't need to be on a waiting list for a kidney and can schedule the surgery when it's best for you, your donor, and your surgeon.

Testing and evaluation at the transplant center may take several visits over weeks to months.

Get on the waiting list

If your tests show you can have a transplant, your transplant center will add your name to the waiting list. Wait times can range from a few months to years. Most transplant centers give preference to people who've been on the waiting list the longest. Other factors, such as your age, where you live, and your blood type, may make your wait longer or shorter.

A transplant center can place you on the waiting list for a donor kidney if your kidney function is 20 or less—even if you aren't on dialysis. While you wait for a kidney transplant, you may need to start dialysis.

Have monthly blood tests

While you wait for a kidney, you'll need monthly blood tests. The center must have a recent sample of your blood to match with any kidney that becomes available.

Have your kidney transplant

During kidney transplant surgery, a surgeon places a healthy kidney into your body. You'll receive general anesthesia before the surgery. The surgery usually takes 3 or 4 hours. Unless your damaged kidneys cause infections or high blood pressure or are cancerous, they can stay in your body. Surgeons usually transplant a kidney into the lower abdomen near the groin.

If you're on a waiting list for a donor kidney, you must go to the hospital to have your transplant surgery as soon as you learn that a kidney is available.

If a family member or friend is donating the kidney, you'll schedule the surgery in advance. Your surgical team will operate on you and your donor at the same time, usually in side-by-side rooms. One surgeon will remove the kidney from the donor, while another prepares you to receive the donated kidney.

Who is on my transplant team?

A successful transplant involves working closely with your transplant team. Members of the team include:

- You—you are an important part of your transplant team.
- Your family members—this may include your spouse, parents, children or any other family member you would like to involve.
- Transplant surgeon—the doctor who places the kidney in your body.
- Nephrologist—a doctor who specializes in kidney health and may work closely with a nurse practitioner or a physician's assistant.
- Transplant coordinator—a specially trained nurse who will be your point of contact, arrange your appointments, and teach you what to do before and after the transplant.

- Pharmacist—a person who tells you about all your medicines, fills your prescriptions, and helps you avoid unsafe medicine combinations and side effects.
- Social worker—a person trained to help you solve problems in your daily life and coordinate care needs after your transplant.
- Dietitian—an expert in food and nutrition who teaches you about the foods you should eat and avoid, and how to plan healthy meals.

Your transplant team will be able to provide the support and encouragement you need throughout the transplant process.

How will I feel after my transplant?

Many people report feeling much better right after having transplant surgery. For some people, it takes a few days for the new kidney to start working.

You probably will need to stay in the hospital several days to recover from surgery—longer if you have any problems after the transplant. You'll have regular follow-up visits with your nephrologist after leaving the hospital.

If you have a living donor, the donor will probably also stay in the hospital for several days. However, a new technique for removing a kidney for donation that uses a smaller cut may make it possible for the donor to leave the hospital in 2 to 3 days.

Before you leave the hospital, you need to learn how to stay healthy and take care of your donor kidney. You will have to take one or more anti-rejection medicines —also called immunosuppressants. Without medicine, your immune system may treat your donor kidney as foreign, or not your own, and attack your new kidney. Anti-rejection medicines may have side effects.

You may also need to take other medicines—for example, antibiotics to protect against infections. Your transplant team will teach you what each medicine is for and when to take each one. Be sure you understand the instructions for taking your medicines before you leave the hospital.

How do I know my new kidney is working?

Blood tests help you know your donor kidney is working. Before you leave the hospital, you'll schedule an appointment at the transplant center to test your blood. The tests show how well your kidneys are removing wastes from your blood.

At first, you'll need regular checkups and blood tests at the transplant center or from your doctor. As time goes on, you'll have fewer checkups.

Your blood tests may show that your kidney is not removing wastes from your blood as well as it should.

You also may have other symptoms that your body is rejecting your donor kidney. If you have these problems, your transplant surgeon or nephrologist may order a kidney biopsy.

What are the possible problems after a kidney transplant?

The donated kidney may start working right away or may take up to a few weeks to make urine. If the new kidney doesn't start working right away, you'll need dialysis treatments to filter wastes and extra salt and fluid from your body until it starts working.

Other problems following kidney transplant are similar to other pelvic surgeries and may include:

- bleeding
- infection, especially a bladder infection
- hernia
- pain or numbness along the inner thigh that usually goes away without treatment

Transplant rejection is rare right after surgery and can take days or weeks to occur. Rejection is less common when the new kidney is from a living donor than when it's from a deceased donor.

What are the symptoms of transplant rejection?

Transplant rejection often begins before you feel any changes. The routine blood tests that you have at the transplant center will reveal early signs of rejection. You may develop high blood pressure or notice swelling because your kidney isn't getting rid of extra salt and fluid in your body.

Your health care provider will treat early signs of rejection by adjusting your medicines to help keep your body from rejecting your new kidney.

Transplant rejection is becoming less common. However, your body may still reject the donor kidney, even if you do everything you should. If that happens, you may need to go on dialysis and go back on the waiting list for another kidney. Some people are able to get a second kidney transplant.

Seek medical care right away

When you're taking anti-rejection medicines, you're at a greater risk for infection. Anti-rejection medicines can dull symptoms of problems such as infection. Call your transplant center right away if you aren't feeling well or have :

- a fever of more than 100 degrees
- drainage from your surgical scar
- burning when you pass urine
- a cold or cough that won't go away

What are the side effects of anti-rejection medicines?

Some anti-rejection medicines may change your appearance. Your face may get fuller, you may gain weight, or you may develop acne or facial hair. Not all people have these side effects.

Anti-rejection medicines weaken your immune system, which can lead to infections. In some people over long periods of time, a weakened immune system can increase their risk of developing cancer. Some anti-rejection medicines cause cataracts, diabetes, extra stomach acid, high blood pressure, and bone disease.

When used over time, these medicines may also cause liver or kidney damage in some people. Your transplant team will order regular tests to monitor the levels of anti-rejection medicines in your blood and to measure your liver and kidney function.

What should I eat or avoid eating with a kidney transplant?

You have more choices about what to eat after you receive a kidney transplant than you would if you were on dialysis. However, you will need to work with a dietitian to develop an eating plan that is best for you.

How do I pay for my transplant?

Medicare, the Federal Government health insurance program, will pay for transplant and care for 3 years after the transplant. Medicare will also pay for your donor's surgery and his or her care. Medicare and private insurance may help pay for your medicines. Additionally, drug companies give discounts to people who can show that they can't afford to pay for their prescriptions. Talk with your transplant social worker to find out what resources are available to help you pay for your transplant.

www.ingramcontent.com/pod-product-compliance
Lightning Source LLC
Chambersburg PA
CBHW031514150726
47990CB00007B/3013